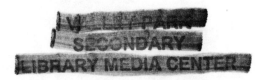

Everything You Need to Know About

Migraines and Other Headaches

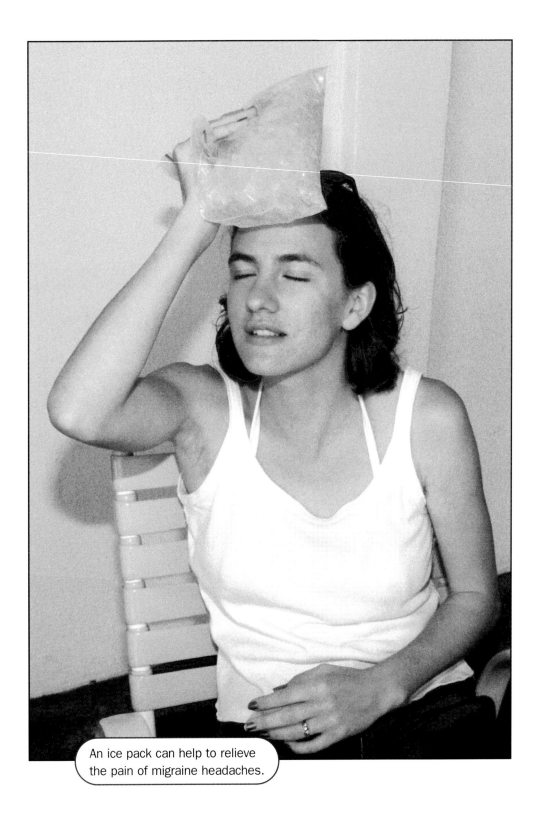

An ice pack can help to relieve the pain of migraine headaches.

Everything You Need to Know About

Migraines and Other Headaches

Barbara Moe

The Rosen Publishing Group, Inc.
New York

Many thanks to Paul G. Moe, M.D., and Alan Seay, M.D., pediatric neurologists at The Children's Hospital in Denver, Colorado; and to Steven L. Lindner, M.D., pediatric neurologist of Dallas Pediatric Neurologists in Dallas, Texas. Thanks also to Cathy LeGrand, librarian at The Children's Hospital of Denver, to David Moe, and to the staff of the Denver Public Library.

Published in 2000 by The Rosen Publishing Group, Inc.
29 East 21st Street, New York, NY 10010

First Edition

Library of Congress Cataloging-in-Publication Data

Moe, Barbara.
  Everything you need to know about migraines and other headaches / Barbara Moe.
     p. cm. — (The need to know library)
  Includes bibliographical references and index.
  Summary: Describes the symptoms, treatment, and prevention of migraine headaches and compares them to other kinds of headaches.
  ISBN 0-8239-3291-5
     1. Migraine—Juvenile literature. [1. Migraine. 2. Headache.]
  I. Title. II. Series.
  RC392 .M64 2000
  616.8'57—dc21
                             00-026927

Manufactured in the United States of America

Contents

Introduction: What Are
    Migraine Headaches?   6

Chapter One   Classifying Migraine
    Headaches   11

Chapter Two   When Headaches Are Not
    Migraines   20

Chapter Three   Recognizing Migraine
    Headaches   28

Chapter Four   Prevention   38

Chapter Five   Treatment and Relief   50

    Glossary   56

    Where to Go for Help   58

    For Further Reading   61

    Index   63

Introduction: What Are Migraine Headaches?

"*I'm the youngest of four kids in our family, and the only one, except my mom, who gets migraines,*" says Maria. "*Sometimes I wake up with it—it's like a knife in my eye. I just want to go back to sleep, but my mom makes me get up and go to school. I sit on the bus with my head between my knees and I press on my eye. I take aspirin or ibuprofen as soon as I can, but sometimes nothing helps. When I get off the bus, I can almost hear the pain beating in my eye.*

"*I don't always wake up with it, and I'm not sure what brings it on. Strong smells can do it, so I tell my friends, 'For my birthday, don't give me perfume. Just send me a card!'*"

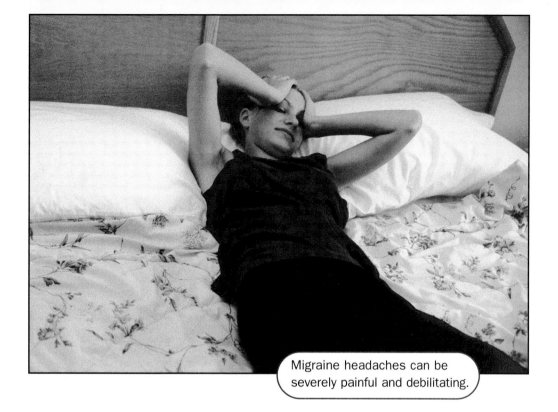

Migraine headaches can be severely painful and debilitating.

What Is Migraine?

Migraine is a condition of recurring severe headaches that are often accompanied by nausea and vomiting. People usually call them "migraine headaches" or simply "migraines." In this book, that is what we will call them, too.

"It's totally weird," says Rob. "My headache hasn't even started yet, but I've already lost my appetite. That's very unusual for me. When this happens I say to myself, 'Uh-oh, headache time.' But I usually don't recognize it soon enough to take pain medication. This is how my headaches often start."

A migraine is not just a bad headache, but a certain type of headache. True migraines do not happen every day. Some people get a migraine only once or twice a year. Other people have migraines as often as ten times a month. In adults, migraine pain is usually on one side of the head, but in kids it is often on both sides. During the migraine, the person may be sensitive to lights and noise.

How Common Are Migraines?

Experts say that twenty-four million Americans (eighteen million women and six million men) get migraine headaches. Up to 90 percent of young people get headaches now and then. Between 4 and 10 percent of these headaches are migraines. This number may be an underestimate, because many people take over-the-counter pain relievers for migraines—or simply suffer.

"I don't suffer in silence," Jake says. "I go around holding a chunk of ice on my head. Or I ask my girlfriend to give me a massage. Nothing really helps, but I need to know someone is there for me. I need sympathy!"

At What Age Do Migraine Headaches Start?

Migraine headaches may start as early as age two or even younger. The frequency of migraines tends to

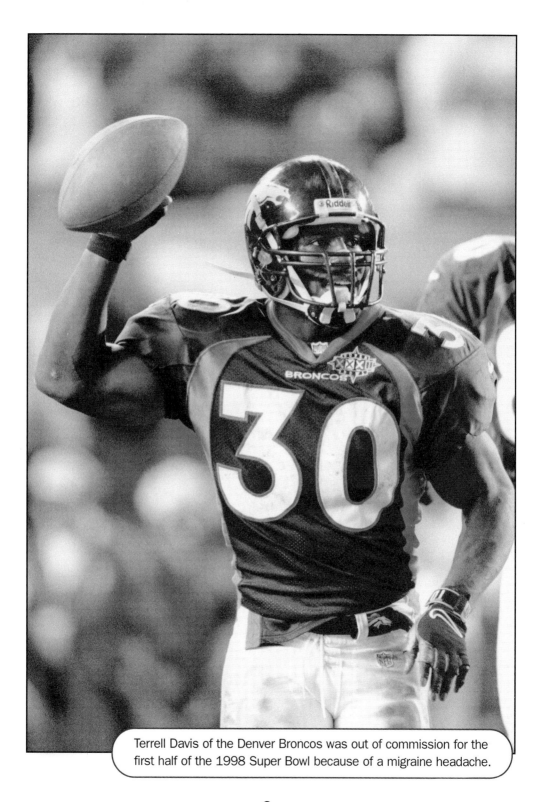

Terrell Davis of the Denver Broncos was out of commission for the first half of the 1998 Super Bowl because of a migraine headache.

peak during the teen years and early twenties. Another peak occurs in people between the ages of thirty-five and forty-five. The older people get, the less likely they are to have migraine attacks.

Who Gets More Migraines—Guys or Girls?

In their early years, boys and girls get migraine headaches in about equal numbers. But after puberty, young women pull ahead. Experts believe hormonal changes related to a woman's menstrual cycle trigger migraine headaches. That is one explanation for women having three times as many headaches as men.

Migraine Equivalents

Cyclic or repeated vomiting, without any headache at all, may be a variety of migraine or a migraine equivalent. Dizziness, vertigo (the feeling that you or your surroundings are tilting or twirling), nausea, vomiting, and abdominal pain can all occur without a headache. Children or young people with migraine equivalents may discover that as they get older, they experience regular migraine headaches.

Chapter One | Classifying Migraine Headaches

One of the weird things about migraine headaches is that what happens *before* the headache may be almost as important as the headache itself. Why? There are two main reasons:

1) Knowing what comes before the headache helps doctors to classify and treat the headache.

2) Various kinds of pain medication are more effective if a person takes these medications as soon as possible—before the headache takes hold.

What May Happen Before a Migraine Begins

The word *prodrome* describes the stage before a headache—the warning period. As much as a day or more before a headache, some young people describe feelings that may be warnings of an oncoming headache, such as irritability, tiredness, and depression.

The Aura

The aura is another experience that occurs even closer to the onset of migraine (thirty to sixty minutes prior). The word *aura* means a sensation of something more to come. Only about 20 percent of those with migraine headaches have auras, but an aura can be as dramatic as fireworks on the Fourth of July.

Auras are often highly visual. People see flashing lights, shimmering or zig-zagging lines, or blind spots. The "Alice-in-Wonderland" syndrome describes visual problems in which large figures turn into small ones and small ones into large. Some people experience numbness or tingling in various parts of their bodies during an aura. Others have trouble speaking.

Two Main Categories of Migraine

In 1988, the International Headache Society decided on two major migraine classifications: migraine without aura—the most common type of migraine—and migraine with aura. In trying to classify your headache and make an accurate diagnosis, your doctor will probably ask you the following questions:

♦ Over a period of time, have you had at least five of these attacks?

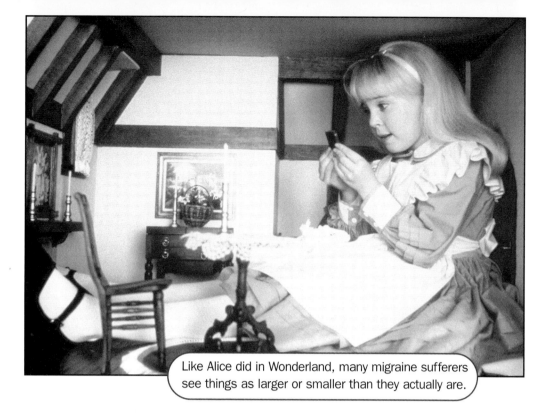

Like Alice did in Wonderland, many migraine sufferers see things as larger or smaller than they actually are.

- Have the headaches lasted from four hours to three days? (In young people a migraine headache may be as short as an hour.)

The doctor's next questions will have to do with how the headache feels to you.

- Is the headache on one side only? (The answer for adult migraine sufferers will likely be "yes," but for young people a migraine headache may be on both sides.)

- Does the headache pound or pulsate?

- Is the headache very painful? In other words, on a scale of 1 to 10, is it at least an 8, 9, or 10?

- Does it hurt more with physical activity?

For a doctor to consider your headache a migraine, the answer would have to be "yes" to at least two of the above questions. A doctor's next set of questions will concern other physical feelings that go along with migraine headaches.

- When you have a headache, do you feel sick to your stomach? Do you throw up?

- During the headache, are you sensitive to lights or noise?

Those who have true migraines will answer "yes" to one or both of the above questions. If you have migraines with aura, mention the sensations you experience to your doctor. An accurate classification of your type of migraine will make treatment more effective.

More Migraine Categories

Some uncommon headaches are even more complicated than those already mentioned. These rare headaches not only hurt but can cause symptoms that can be very scary.

Basilar Artery Migraine

These headaches are most likely to affect teenage women. The sufferer may vomit, experience visual problems, dizziness, vertigo, trouble walking, and even loss of consciousness. Unlike the usual migraine headache, this one may hurt in the back of the head.

14

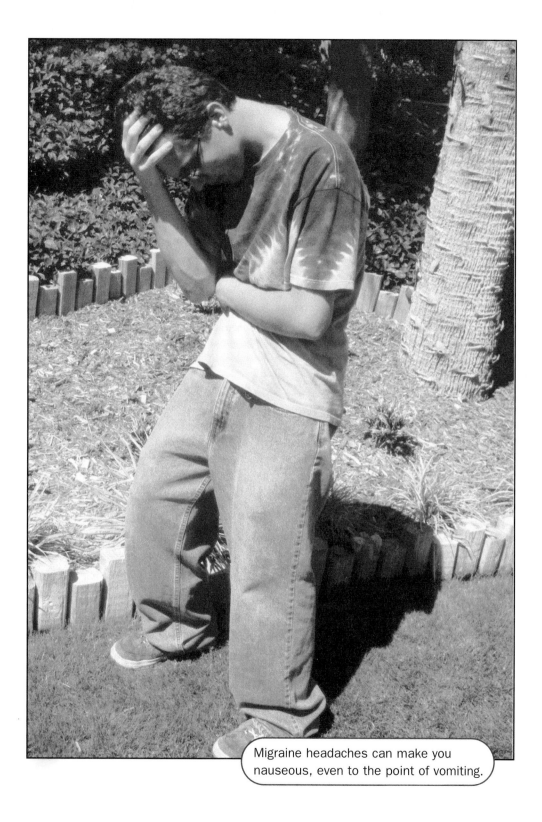

Migraine headaches can make you nauseous, even to the point of vomiting.

Hemiplegic Migraine

Scientists have found specific genetic markers for this type of headache. That is why it is sometimes called *familial* hemiplegic migraine. The hemiplegia (paralysis of one side of the body) or hemiparesis (weakness of one side of the body) at the onset of this headache sometimes lasts well after the headache ends.

Confusional Migraine

A confused mental state, including possible amnesia, is the hallmark of the confusional migraine, which is more common in boys. The sufferer may become restless and disoriented. Afterward, he or she may have no memory of the headache.

> *In PE class, Tyler felt a headache coming on. Then his legs became numb. The numbness spread to his left arm, and he couldn't move his fingers. Next, he couldn't talk. He started to see what looked like sparklers. When he became confused and disoriented, the school nurse called an ambulance. In the emergency room at the hospital, Tyler vomited twice. All diagnostic tests came out normal, however, and eight hours later Tyler felt fine.*

Ophthalmoplegic Migraine

The double vision and other eye problems that accompany this rare headache may last a long time after the headache is gone.

16

Cluster Headache

Another rare variety of headache is the cluster headache. Some say it is a migraine and some say it isn't,
but people describe it as extremely painful. However, it
rarely appears in people under twenty.

What Causes Migraine Headaches?

Scientists believe that migraine headaches have strong
genetic roots. At least 70 percent of those with
migraine headaches have a close relative (usually a par-
ent or grandparent) who also has migraines.

Although no one knows the exact mechanism, it
appears that those who get migraines have a mild insta-
bility of the nervous system and blood vessels. During a
migraine attack, a "spreading depression" of tiny elec-
trical currents travels from the back to the front of the
brain. This current can cause the blood vessels in the
brain to tighten and deliver less blood. The migraine sufferer may experience an aura, blurry vision, or dizziness
from this partial blood shutdown. When the blood vessels rebound, they dilate, or swell up. This may cause
them to leak a small amount of pain-causing chemicals
into the skin of the scalp.

The structures in the head that can hurt are the
nerves, the blood vessels, and the covering of the
brain, not the brain itself. A large nerve (the fifth, or
trigeminal, nerve) on the underside of the brain senses

chemical and blood vessel changes. At the same time, serotonin, a neurotransmitter that carries messages from nerve to nerve, is also involved in the transmission of pain. A lack of serotonin can make the blood vessels swell or become larger, causing the throbbing pain of a migraine.

Migraine Myths

You may have heard things about the causes of migraine that are not true. Remember that when you talk about having a "migraine," you are talking about a specific *type* of headache, not just an aching head. The following are some common myths about migraines.

Myth: Sinus trouble causes migraine headaches.

Fact: A sinus infection may cause a headache, but probably not a migraine.

Myth: Eye strain causes migraine headaches.

Fact: Eye strain is unlikely to cause migraine headaches or other headaches.

Myth: Allergies cause migraine headaches.

Fact: A migraine headache is not an allergic reaction, and allergies are rarely a cause of migraine headaches.

Myth: If you get a lot of migraine headaches, you probably have a brain tumor.

Fact: Brain tumors cause a very small percentage of headaches. Also, migraine headaches occur in cycles. A brain tumor usually causes a headache that gets progressively worse over time.

In short, headaches manifest themselves in many ways. The more information you can provide your doctor about the circumstances in which you experience the headache, and the other symptoms occurring with it, the more easily your doctor can diagnose the type of headache you are experiencing. Then he or she can suggest appropriate treatment.

Chapter Two | **When Headaches Are Not Migraines**

People who have frequent headaches often have more than one type of headache. Sometimes one kind of headache merges into another.

Last Halloween, Lisa had a tension headache. She remembers it well because it felt as if she was carrying a twenty-five pound pumpkin on her head. By the next day, the pain had moved to her eye socket and began to throb. The nurse at school said that Lisa's headache was probably a migraine. On Christmas Day, Lisa got another migraine that hurt more than any headache she had ever had. That one turned into a chronic daily headache, which didn't go away completely until school started in January.

Like Lisa, some people have a combination of migraine and tension headaches. They find it hard to figure out where one headache ends and the other begins.

Cedric thinks that the stress connected with this year's Homecoming Dance may have contributed to the stabbing head pain that hit him in the middle of the dance. Luckily, he made it to the men's room in time to throw up. He had drunk two cups of coffee at the pre-dinner party and two more during dinner. Cedric had already identified caffeine as one of his headache triggers. Why did he do this to himself?

He felt fine the next day, but every day for the next week he had a dull headache. It seemed to get worse during his fourth-period math class. On a scale of 1 to 10, Cedric gave his migraine a 10. He gave his tension headache a 5 or a 6.

Tension Headaches

Most headaches are not migraines. Probably the most common of all headaches is the tension headache. People used to call tension headaches stress headaches or muscle-contraction headaches. Although stress may play a role in the development of a tension headache, it is not the only cause.

Tension headaches often feel as if a belt or a piece of elastic has been pulled tightly around the scalp.

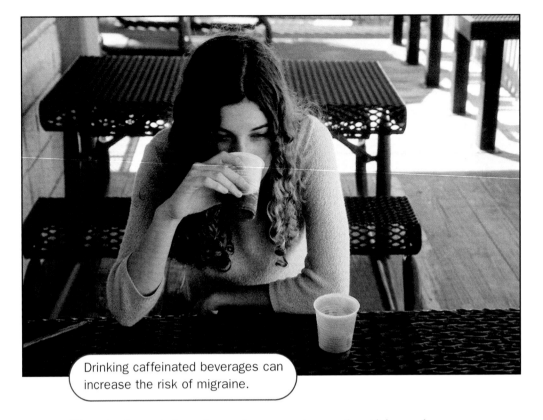

Drinking caffeinated beverages can increase the risk of migraine.

Physical activity doesn't seem to make this pain any worse. The head doesn't throb as it would with a migraine, and the person doesn't usually vomit or feel nauseated. When a tension headache makes the person sensitive to bright lights and certain noises, it may be hard to distinguish from a migraine. In fact, some researchers believe that tension headaches are a less intense form of migraine. The headache can last from one hour to several days. Doctors classify tension headaches in two ways:

Episodic Tension Headaches

"Episodic" means repeatedly, or happening over and over. A doctor may classify your headaches in this category if you experience a couple of headaches most weeks but fewer than fifteen episodes a month. Most people with episodic tension headaches get relief from over-the-counter pain medications, ice packs to the head, naps, and/or relaxation exercises.

Chronic Tension Headaches/Chronic Daily Headaches

Imagine having a headache every day of your life. This kind of pain can really get to you. Those with chronic daily headaches have discomfort every day (or almost every day) for six months or longer. Over-the-counter pain relievers do not help. In fact, some pain medications can even make a headache worse, causing a "rebound headache." A person with any kind of headache who takes too much pain medication can experience the rebound syndrome. When this happens, it is recommended that sufferers stop taking all pain medications.

Serious Headaches

We can divide headaches other than tension headaches into two categories, according to the cause, and whether or not the cause is life-threatening. Chances are you will never experience the causes of these types of headaches. They are serious but rare.

Brain Tumors

Brain tumors cause many of the same symptoms as migraines. But over time, a brain-tumor headache will

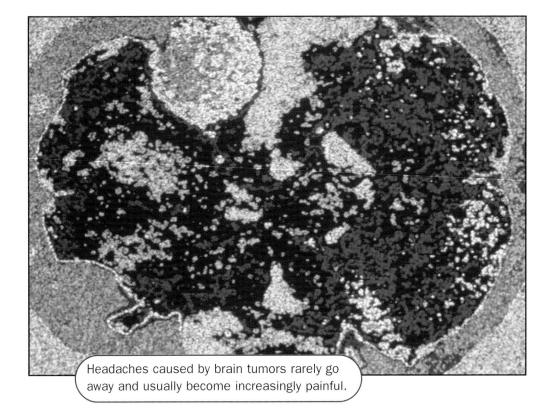

Headaches caused by brain tumors rarely go away and usually become increasingly painful.

hurt more, last longer, and is not likely to go away. If you have never had a serious headache and suddenly experience this kind of pain, you should see a doctor right away. A headache accompanied by seizures, vomiting, or troubles with balance should be checked out.

Remember again that brain tumors are rare. Also, a brain tumor is not a death sentence. After treatment with surgery, chemotherapy, and/or radiation, many people with brain tumors go on to lead normal lives.

Meningitis
Meningitis is an inflammation of the membrane (meninges) that surrounds the brain and spinal cord. A bacteria or a virus causes this infection. One of the main

symptoms of meningitis is a stiff neck. Other symptoms are a bad headache that doesn't go away, fever, lack of energy, or unconsciousness. Bacterial meningitis can be very serious, but treatment with specialized antibiotics usually cures the disease. Viral meningitis is usually not as serious as bacterial meningitis.

Aneurysm

An aneurysm is a bulging or weak blood vessel. When an aneurysm leaks or bursts, it causes a hemorrhage, or severe bleeding. If a hemorrhage goes into or around the brain, the bleeding will cause great pain (a thunderclap headache). Also, as with meningitis, the bleeding will cause a stiff neck. If not treated by surgery, the aneurysm may cause unconsciousness or even death.

Severe Head Injury/Subdural Bleeding

A severe head injury from an accident, fall, or from physical abuse can also cause bleeding in the head. This can result in a bad headache. Subdural bleeding occurs between the underside of the skull and the brain. A surgeon will have to drain the hemorrhage. This condition is a medical emergency.

Less Serious Headaches

Exertional Headaches

Exertion includes any kind of physical activity, even coughing. Exertion can cause headaches in some people.

Altitude Headaches

Until they become accustomed to the thinner air, people who go to places at high altitudes may experience headaches. Exertion, such as hiking or skiing, may make the headache worse. Altitude headaches cause a throbbing, pulsating pain. Pain relievers and increased oxygen sometimes help, but the best way to get rid of an altitude headache is to go back down the mountain.

Influenza and Other Viral or Bacterial Illnesses

Headaches often go hand-in-hand with various infections and fever. Bacteria and viruses produce headache-causing toxins (poisons). Fever can also cause headaches because of the increased blood flow to the brain and the dilation of the blood vessels.

Headaches From Substances

Some headaches are caused by ingesting or being exposed to certain substances. One common headache-causing food is ice cream. However, an ice cream headache usually lasts only a few minutes.

Drugs can cause much worse and longer-lasting headaches. Some of the drugs likely to cause headaches include alcohol, cocaine, and marijuana. Drinking too much alcohol causes many people to wake up the next morning with throbbing head pain. Drugs that raise the body's metabolism and blood pressure, such as cocaine, can even cause an aneurysm.

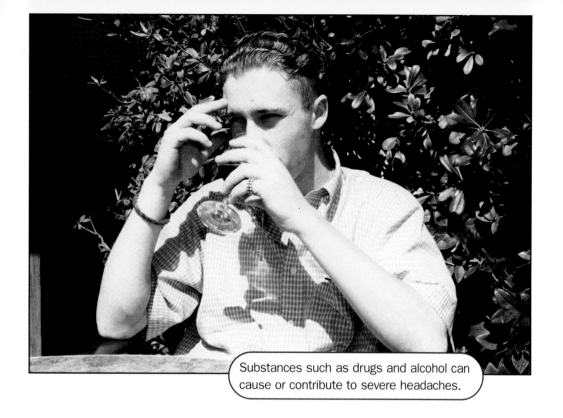

Substances such as drugs and alcohol can cause or contribute to severe headaches.

Carbon monoxide, often caused by leaking heaters or gas stoves, can also cause headaches. This headache can be a warning of danger to come. If the level of carbon monoxide in a person's blood rises to over 50 percent, the person may go into coma and die. For protection, your family should have a carbon monoxide detector installed in your home.

Chapter Three

Recognizing Migraine Headaches

Headaches are scary. Headaches interfere with your life. Headaches make you depressed. However, the more you know about your headaches, the better you will be able to deal with them. Steve Lindner, M.D., a pediatric neurologist in Dallas, Texas, says that most kids want to know three things about their headaches:

- What is the cause?
- What will make my headaches better?
- Are you sure I don't have a life-threatening illness?

Most people don't go to the doctor if they feel they don't have to. Even those with the most severe headaches tend to treat themselves with over-the-counter pain medications, or just suffer. But when headaches start to interfere with your life, you need to get help.

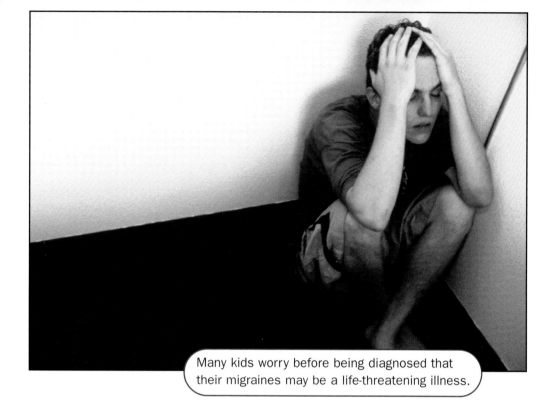

Many kids worry before being diagnosed that their migraines may be a life-threatening illness.

Who Can Help?

Medical Practitioners

As we have seen, medical conditions can contribute to headaches. When your head feels ready to pop, you want instant relief, but first you should find out the cause of your headaches. Medical practitioners are the best-equipped professionals to figure out your headache type and to offer appropriate remedies.

Primary Care Physicians

Your primary care physician may be a general practitioner, a family physician, a pediatrician, or even an emergency room doctor. It is helpful if this doctor is someone you have known over the years and feel comfortable with. If your primary doctor can diagnose and treat your headaches, you may not have to see a specialist.

Specialists

If, after a period of time, you do not get relief from your headaches, you may need to see a specialist. Your primary physician can refer you to a pediatric neurologist, who is a specialist in two disciplines: pediatrics (the care of young people) and neurology (the care of the brain, spinal cord, and nerves).

In addition to a primary doctor and/or a neurologist, you may also get help from a psychologist or psychiatrist. Both specialize in the ways emotions contribute to physical illness, and the ways in which physical illnesses contribute to emotional distress. For example, a person who has frequent, severe migraines or chronic daily headaches may get depressed and feel that life with a constant headache is not worth living.

"I used to be a very outgoing person," says Sienna. "But my headaches turned me into a hermit. I always felt sick to my stomach, so going out to eat didn't work. When I had a migraine, I didn't want to move at all because that made my head throb. The only thing I ever wanted to do was sleep. Eventually, my friends stopped calling me. When my doctor suggested I see a psychologist, I

was sort of skeptical, but I went. I started taking medication and made some lifestyle changes too. Today, I rarely have to see any doctors. I can truly say I'm a new woman!"

Psychologists and licensed clinical social workers can help manage your depressive feelings and stress. Psychiatrists are counselors, too. In addition, psychiatrists can prescribe medication to treat depression. A children's hospital or university hospital may also have a headache clinic. If you go to a headache clinic, your doctor will be a specialist who sees people with the most stubborn and hard-to-treat headaches.

The Doctor Takes the History

One of the most important things a doctor does before making a diagnosis of migraine or other headache is to take a history. Your parents have known you your whole life, and they also know about their own parents. Because migraines tend to run in families, try to get both of your parents to go with you on your first visit to the doctor. However, if there are things that you would like to discuss in privacy, it's okay to ask to speak to the doctor alone.

In chapter 1 we went over some questions doctors ask to help them classify headaches. Before doing a physical examination, the doctor will ask more questions.

Family and Social History

- Who else in your family (on your mother's or father's side) has had migraines or other headaches? Do either of your parents have migraines? Do any of your siblings have headaches?

- Are any past or current events causing you extreme grief—death, divorce, family turmoil, trouble in school or with friends?

- Have you had any significant illness? Are you taking any regular medications, drinking alcohol, or using any illegal substances?

Your Personal Headache History

- How old do you think you were when you had your first headache?

- Have your headaches gotten better or worse since that first one?

- Have you noticed anything that seems to trigger a headache? A certain food? Bright light? Stress? Menstrual periods?

- At what time of day do you usually get a headache?

- What have you tried to cure your headaches? What works? What doesn't work?

- Are you worried about a more serious cause of your headaches, such as illness?

The Physical Exam

The physical exam is important because it can rule out serious headache causes. A doctor will look in your eyes and test your balance and reflexes. These observations can tell a great deal about what is (or what is not) going on in your brain. Keep in mind that a doctor does everything for a reason. If a physician asks you to hop on one foot, he or she is not trying to find out if you would make a good cheerleader. The goal is to discover if your brain, nerves, and muscles are working correctly. If a neurologist pricks your skin, it is to check your nerve functions, not to cause you pain.

Other Diagnostic Tools

CT Scan

CT (computed tomography) scans are also called CAT (computerized axial tomography) scans. These are fancy names for taking a picture of your brain. A neuro-imaging system allows doctors to map cross-sections of various parts of your body, including your brain. Scans are useful in detecting tumors, hemorrhages, and other serious causes of headaches.

MRI and MRA

Magnetic resonance imaging (MRI) and magnetic resonance angiography (MRA) are both painless picture-taking procedures. The MRI uses powerful magnets to detect serious brain abnormalities, such as tumors and hemorrhages. The MRA (magnetic resonance angiography) is a similar procedure used to observe the large blood vessels of the head to see if there are abnormalities or obstructions.

Angiography

Angiography is a more invasive procedure than MRI or MRA. A doctor inserts a small tube into a blood vessel. The tube is used to insert a dye into the blood vessel that shows if there has been a rupture. In many situations, MRIs and MRAs have replaced angiography.

Electroencephalogram (EEG)

An EEG is usually not a part of a doctor's study of headaches. It is a painless procedure in which electrodes, attached to a patient's scalp, show unusual brain wave patterns.

Lumbar Puncture (LP)

A lumbar puncture or spinal tap, as it is sometimes called, is not necessary in routine headache testing. Its major use is in diagnosing meningitis (infection of the linings of the brain) or encephalitis (infection of the brain itself).

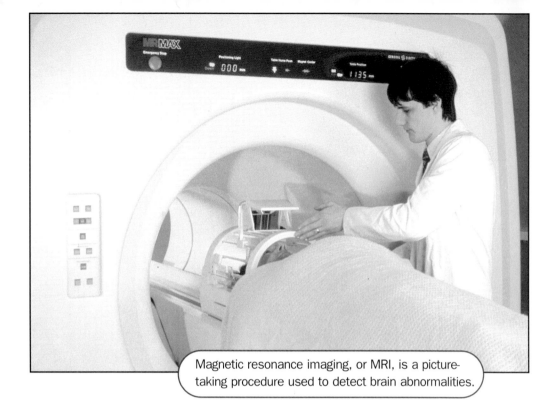

Magnetic resonance imaging, or MRI, is a picture-taking procedure used to detect brain abnormalities.

How You Can Help

As you may have guessed, reporting your condition honestly to your doctor is one of the most important parts of the migraine diagnosis.

Tell Your Headache Story

Now that you know some of the questions a doctor will ask, keep these questions in mind. Write down your "headache story." Make sure that the story you write down is honest. The personal story of your headaches, including when they started and what they are like, will be very helpful to the doctor who is trying to diagnose you. Be sure to bring your story to your first doctor visit.

Draw A Picture Of Your Headache

Think back to your most recent headache. Was it unusually bad? Can you remember the worst headache you ever had? Do you have a headache right now? Try to draw how it feels. Where does it hurt? How much does it hurt? What color is it? Make some labels to go with your picture. Draw cartoons. Take your pictures to your doctor. You will be surprised how much he or she will appreciate it.

Your Headache Diary

The idea of a diary devoted exclusively to your headaches may not appeal to you. Some headaches are so bad that you wonder how you could ever forget them. But as one headache merges into another, you may not remember as much as you expect. Do you remember exactly what stressed you on Monday, or when you ate chocolate on Tuesday? The answer to a memory problem is a precise headache diary.

Some doctors will give you a headache diary with a formatted table, but you can also design your own pages. Get a loose-leaf notebook and fill it with paper, or make up a form on your computer. Below are some categories that you might want to include.

- Day and date
- When headache began and ended

- Warning signs

- Other symptoms

- Medications taken

- Things that helped you feel better

- Location of headache

- Type of pain

- Intensity of pain on a scale of 1 to 10

- What you ate or drank pre-headache

- Unusual events or stressors

Keep your headache diary as faithfully as you can and for as long as you can. Be sure to take your headache diary to your doctor. Together, the two of you can try to find headache patterns and contributing factors.

Honesty Is The Best Policy

Above all, be honest with yourself and your doctor.

> *"I was missing school because of headaches,"* says Natasha. *"When the doctor asked me—right in front of my mom—about drinking alcohol, I said, 'Oh, I don't drink!' Yeah, right. I was drinking every weekend and staying up half the night. No wonder I had headaches."*

Chapter Four

Prevention

When it comes to headache prevention, there is good news and bad news. The bad news is that preventing your headaches may not be entirely possible. The good news is that prevention is definitely worth a try. Work on the lifestyle changes listed below. They won't hurt and they may help. (Medications for headache prevention are listed last, because doctors prescribe them only for frequent and stubborn headaches.)

Avoiding Headache Triggers

Various influences combine to produce a headache. Headache "triggers" are internal or external forces that contribute to migraine in susceptible people. One person's triggers may not even bother another person. The goal is to determine your personal triggers.

TRIGGERS

These are some of the most common headache triggers.

Dietary Triggers

Beer, wine (especially red), and hard alcohol

Aspartame (Nutrasweet)

Avocados

Bananas

Caffeine, especially in large amounts

Cheese, such as brie, cheddar, and mozzarella

Chocolate and cocoa

Coffee

Dairy products, such as sour cream, yogurt, and milk

Fruits, especially citrus, such as lemons, limes, and oranges

Monosodium glutamate (MSG)

Nitrites, used in preserving foods such as bacon, bologna, hot dogs, and pepperoni

Nuts and seeds

Olive oil

Onions

Peanut butter

Soft drinks

Tea

Environmental Triggers

Air pollution

Altitude changes

Light, such as bright sunlight, light from movie and computer screens, or flashing lights

Noise, especially loud and constant sounds

Odors, such as those from perfume, cigarette smoke, or chemicals

Weather-related factors, such as wind, humidity, or thunderstorms

Personal Triggers

Anxiety

Depression

Emotional turmoil, such as relationship problems, divorce, or a death in the family

Exertion, such as too much exercise or heavy lifting

Irregular eating habits, such as skipping meals

Menstrual cycle

Medications, such as the antibiotic tetracycline

Sleep (too much or too little)

Stress and tension

Travel, especially across time zones

Some experts say the role of triggers in migraine headaches is overemphasized. Others disagree. They are your headaches, so you be the judge.

Staying in Shape

See if exercising three or four times a week for at least twenty minutes a day boosts your headache-prevention threshold. Running, swimming, and playing basketball are all excellent ways to exercise, and doing activities that you enjoy will make you more likely to continue.

Avoiding Stress

Avoiding stress is easier said than done. In fact, you can't avoid stress completely unless you want to become a hermit. The important thing is how you react to stress.

*"My best friend Kate sort of turned on me,"
says Melanie. "She started telling people that I
was annoying her. I said to myself, 'If I'm irritating her, maybe I'm irritating everyone else, too.' I
lost faith in myself. I got so upset—Kate and I
had been friends since first grade—that I started
getting headaches."*

*Dr. Santos, a psychologist, helped Melanie to
recognize that she had a problem with Kate, not
with herself. She advised Melanie to steer clear of
Kate for a while. "If you're forced into a group
together," said Dr. Santos, "concentrate on your
deep breathing and remove yourself from the sit-
uation as soon as possible." When Kate discovered she could no longer push Melanie's buttons,
she stopped picking on her, and Melanie's headaches went away.*

Learning to Relax

You may have already found your own ways to relax.
Listening to music is one way; talking with friends is
another. Experts also suggest the following techniques.
Try some of them and see if they work for you.

Imagery and/or Visualization

Once a headache has taken hold, it may be too late to
use imagery or visualization. Don't wait for a headache
to practice seeing yourself in a relaxing setting, free of

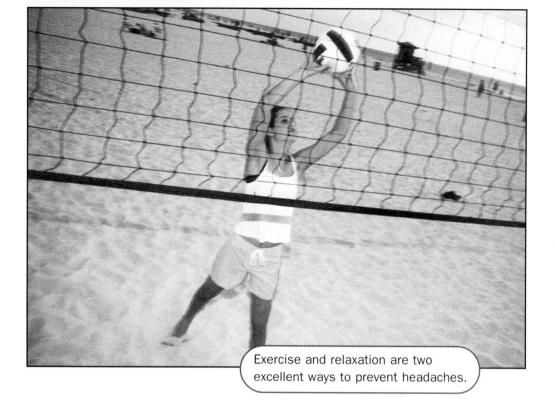

Exercise and relaxation are two excellent ways to prevent headaches.

stress. Close your eyes and imagine yourself on a quiet beach. You hear no sounds, except for the crash of waves against the shore. Inhale. Smell the salty ocean air. Imagine the heat of the sun on your shoulders and the burning sand under your feet. To make visualization even easier, get a tape with relaxing music and directions to guide you.

Conscious Breathing

Breathing is something we do twenty-four hours a day, but we don't usually give it much thought. Try paying attention to your breath. (Concentrating on your breath is one of many types of meditation.) Wearing comfortable clothes, sit in a chair in a quiet place. Inhale and count slowly to three. Exhale. Pay attention only to your breathing. Keep up this conscious inhaling and exhaling for several minutes.

Progressive Muscle Relaxation

Lie on the floor or on a bed. The idea is to squeeze every voluntary muscle in your body, hold the squeeze for a few seconds, and then relax. Start with your head, the source of your misery. Squeeze your eyebrows together into a frown. Hold that pose as long as you can, then relax. Then, squeeze your eyes tightly shut. Relax. Next, scrunch up your nose like a rabbit. Hold it. Relax. Get the idea? Move down your body, tensing and relaxing every muscle you can think of.

Lighten Up!

Studies show that laughter helps to relieve stress. In the middle of a migraine, you may not feel much like laughing. But in your headache-free periods, get in the humor habit. Watch funny movies. Make someone else laugh and laugh with them. Laughing relaxes your face muscles and is good exercise.

Biofeedback

Biofeedback is a painless procedure that uses electronic equipment to measure your body processes. It then "feeds back" the information to you. After you become more aware of some of your autonomic, or involuntary, body processes, you can exercise more control over them.

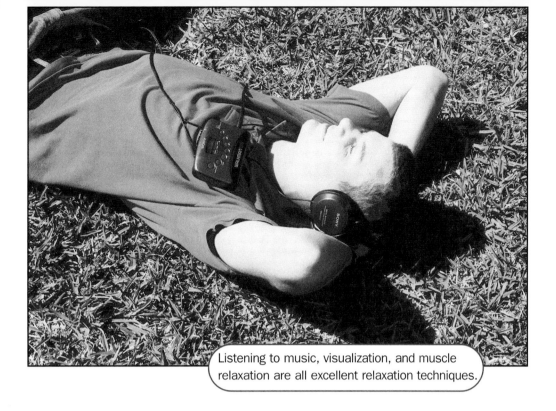

Listening to music, visualization, and muscle relaxation are all excellent relaxation techniques.

If you want to try biofeedback, you will need to go to a biofeedback specialist, who may be a psychologist. He or she will take your headache history. You will have an opportunity to see the machines that record information about your brain waves and skin temperature. After several sessions, you may be able to visualize what happens to you during a migraine. You can then learn how to prevent future migraines.

Yoga

Yoga is a very popular form of relaxation that helps to relieve anxiety and stress. It is an ancient system of exercises, postures, stretches, breathing, and meditation. You can learn yoga in a class or individually with an instructor.

T'ai Chi Chaun (T'ai Chi)

T'ai chi, a Chinese martial art, is also used to relieve stress and to encourage healing. It involves slow, graceful body movements. *Chi* is the Chinese term for the body's vital energy force. You can do t'ai chi by yourself or in a group.

Liking Yourself

If you didn't learn to value yourself as a young child, you may have trouble learning to like yourself now. A therapist (psychiatrist, psychologist, or clinical social worker) will be able to point out some of your self-defeating habits and help you change them for the better. You can also change the way that you view yourself on your own.

- **Affirmations:** Instead of getting down on yourself, as people with chronic headaches tend to do, build yourself up. When you are going to sleep, waking up, walking, or riding in the car, repeat affirmations (positive statements) about yourself. Say them over silently or out loud: "People like me, and I like myself." "I see great things in my future." "With help, I can get control of my headaches."

- **Assertiveness:** Assertiveness training teaches you how to stand up for yourself.

46

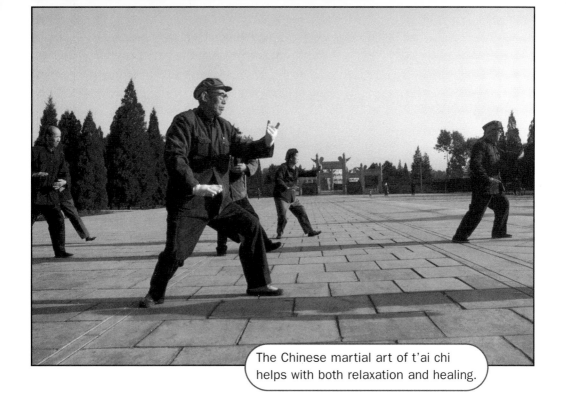

The Chinese martial art of t'ai chi helps with both relaxation and healing.

When sticking up for your rights, you don't have to be obnoxious or loud. Calm firmness will do the trick.

Herbs, Vitamins, and Minerals

If you want to try natural remedies for the prevention of migraines, be sure to check with your doctor first. Excessive doses of some herbal substances can do more harm than good. For example, high doses of Vitamin A can *cause* headaches. Natural may be best for some people, but even natural remedies have a potential for harm. Herbal remedies can cause side effects and may have a negative interaction with other drugs.

Migraine Prevention Medications

Ask yourself these questions:

- Do I have more than two migraine headaches a month?
- Do I have migraines that severely disrupt my life?
- Are the medications I am taking to relieve my headaches ineffective?

If you answered "yes" to any of the questions above, your doctor may be willing to prescribe preventive medications. It is up to you whether or not you want to take a pill every day. Sometimes, after taking preventive medication for about six months or so, your doctor will help you to taper off the medication. Many people are able to stay off it for good.

The following medications are commonly used for young people. They are safe when prescribed by a medical doctor. They are listed with their scientific names first. The trade names are in parentheses.

One migraine prevention drug is an antihistamine called cyproheptadine (Periactin). People usually take this medication at bedtime. Teens sometimes have good luck with small doses of tricyclic antidepressants, such as amitriptyline (Elavil). Another helpful class of preventive drugs are beta blockers. Doctors originally used these medications to control high blood pressure. They help to prevent migraine headaches by stabilizing the blood vessels and regulating blood flow to the brain. Examples of these medications are propranalol (Inderal), nadolol (Corgard), and atenolol (Tenormin).

There is help available for migraine sufferers, and new drugs are appearing every year. Medication, in combination with wellness strategies, can greatly reduce the suffering caused by migraine headaches.

Chapter Five

Treatment and Relief

Just as headaches are divided into categories, so is treatment. We can divide headache treatment into medicinal and nonmedicinal.

Medicinal Migraine Treatment

In considering treatment for your headaches, a doctor may prescribe medicines that will relieve accompanying symptoms as well as the pain in your head. Be sure to start out taking the smallest amount of medication that works.

Nonprescription Medications

A doctor will probably suggest that you first try nonprescription (over-the-counter) medications. Take them at the first sign of a headache. These include aceta-

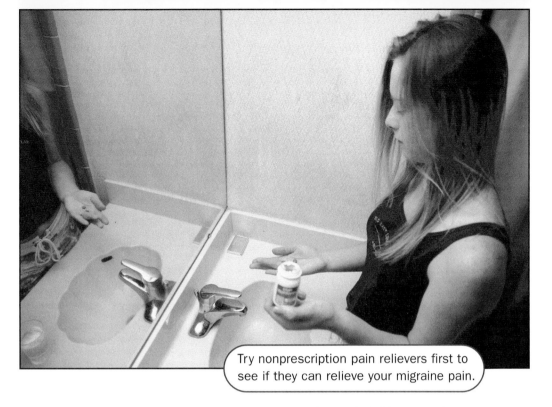

Try nonprescription pain relievers first to see if they can relieve your migraine pain.

minophen (Tylenol) or ibuprofen (Advil, Nuprin, or Motrin). People under the age of fifteen should not use aspirin because of the danger of Reye's syndrome, an illness that causes severe vomiting and possibly coma. Other types of headache relievers are the nonsteroidal anti-inflammatory drugs (NSAIDs). These include naproxen sodium, sold over-the-counter as Aleve.

Prescription Medications

If you need something to relieve the nausea and vomiting caused by your migraines, the doctor may prescribe antiemetics, such as Promethazine (Phenergan) or prochlorperazine (Compazine). Both are available by mouth (for nausea) or by suppository (in case of vomiting). Another antinausea medication is metoclopramide

(Reglan), which is available by mouth or, if necessary, by intravenous injection (IV).

For a full-blown headache, doctors sometimes prescribe a combination drug. Three medications—isometheptene mucate, a vasoactive agent; dichloralphenazone, a nonbarbiturate sedative; and acetaminophen, a painkiller—are all present in Midrin. Fioricet and Esgic are trade names for another combination: acetaminophen for pain relief; butalbitol for sleep; and caffeine.

For teens with severe headaches, doctors may prescribe ergotamine tartrate (Cafergot or Wigraine), a medication that constricts the blood vessels to prevent future blood vessel dilatation. Tablets called Ergomar or Ergostat are available for absorption under the tongue for those who are experiencing vomiting. An ergotamine nasal spray, Migranol, is also available. Sometimes, especially in the emergency room, doctors may use dehydroergotamine (DHE 45) by injection or intravenously.

A blessing for some migraine sufferers is the newer triptan category of medications. One example is sumatriptan (Imitrex), which is available in tablets, by injection, or by nasal spray. Although the nasal spray is effective, it leaves an unpleasant aftertaste. Other triptans include naratriptan (Amerge) and rizatriptan (Maxalt). One drawback is that these new medications are expensive.

Nonmedicinal Treatments

Some methods of migraine treatment are nonmedicinal.

- **Sleep:** Sleep is one of the most effective treatments for migraine headaches. For some people, a nap or a full night's sleep is all that is needed to beat the pain.

- **Ice:** An ice pack on your aching head will probably not cure your headache, but it may make it feel better for a while.

- **Exercise:** Exercise may seem like the opposite of relaxation, but many people find that exercise helps to calm them down. Exercise can make some headaches worse, but for other headaches, exercise is a pain reliever.

- **Massage:** A massage always feels good, especially to those with tension or chronic daily headaches. You don't need a professional massage. Find someone who is willing to rub or knead those oh-so-sore neck and head muscles. Touch is a powerful pain reliever.

- **Individual and Group Therapy:** Psychological therapy won't relieve your headaches completely. But therapy can help to relieve stress and depression, which are frequent contributors to headaches.

Support and Self-Help Groups

Support groups in which you meet other headache sufferers will give you comfort as well as new ideas for headache relief. Your doctor may be able to suggest a local support group. You may also want to join the National Headache Foundation or the American Council for Headache Education. These organizations will give you a list of contacts in your state or will help you start your own support group. If you can't get together with other people, you can get on the Internet and find support on-line. Remember to check out any advice with a medical professional. For helpful organizations and on-line sites in the United States and Canada, see the Where to Go for Help section at the end of this book.

Alternative Treatments

When we talk about treatments for migraines, we are talking about whatever works for you. You may want to seek out alternative treatments. This means that you may want to get treatment outside of a traditional physician's office. However, you could be making a serious mistake if you use only alternative treatments for headaches in the event of a life-threatening cause, such as a brain tumor.

Alternative approaches include acupuncture (the insertion of fine needles through the skin at specific points on the body) and acupressure (the use of pressure points at certain body sites). Other alternative therapies include aromatherapy (the use of aromatic oils to reduce stress), color therapy (the use of colored lights), dance therapy, hydrotherapy (the use of hot and cold water to relieve pain), hypnotherapy (using the unconscious mind to promote healing), and sound therapy (the use of music and other noises).

If you want to learn more about alternative treatments, you can find excellent books on the subject at any public library. Some of these titles are listed in the For Further Reading section at the back of this book.

Hope for the Future

Researchers are making new headache treatments available all the time. Just remember that neither medical science nor alternative practitioners have discovered a headache cure. And yet, with a combination of prevention and treatment methods tailored specifically for you, you can get headache relief.

Glossary

analgesic Drug that relieves pain.

antibiotic Medication that inhibits the growth of microorganisms.

aneurysm Weakness in the wall of a blood vessel that may rupture.

aspartame Powder used as an artificial sweetener, sold under the brand name Nutrasweet.

auras Sensory experiences, such as sparkling lights, that appear for some people thirty to sixty minutes before a migraine headache begins.

encephalitis Inflammation of the brain often caused by a virus.

ergotamine tartrate A vasoconstrictor used in migraine treatment.

headache clinic A center that specializes in the treatment of headaches.

hemiparesis Weakness on one side of the body.

hemiplegia Paralysis on one side of the body.

hemorrhage Severe bleeding.

magnetic resonance imaging (MRI) Procedure that uses a magnetic field and radio waves to detect disease.

meningitis Inflammation of the coverings of the brain.

migraine equivalent Rare type of migraine in which the pain is not in the head but somewhere else, such as in the stomach.

prodrome Early warning period before the onset of a migraine.

subdural Space between the linings over the brain that can fill with blood after an injury.

sublingual Under the tongue.

suppository Medicine in a form that can be inserted into the rectum for absorption.

triggers Anything that sets off a headache, including food, beverages, environmental conditions, psychological stressors, hormonal changes, or changes in one's normal routine.

vertigo A feeling that one's surroundings are tilting or twisting.

Where to Go for Help

In the United States

American Council for Headache Education (ACHE)
19 Mantua Road
Mount Royal, NJ 08061
(800) 255-ACHE
(856) 423-0258
e-mail: achehq@talley.com
Web site: http://www.achenet.org
ACHE is a nonprofit organization that works with patients and doctors to help people participate in their own care. The organization publishes a quarterly newsletter, *Headache;* helps to organize support groups; offers support services on-line.

National Headache Foundation (NHF)
428 West Saint James Place, 2nd Floor
Chicago, IL 60614-2750
(888) NHF-5552
(800) 843-2256
Web site: http://www.headaches.org
The oldest and largest organization for those with headaches, the NHF is a volunteer, nonprofit group that provides free information about headaches, sends out lists of doctors who are members of the foundation, publishes a quarterly newsletter, *NHF Head Lines,* and can provide localized lists of support groups. If there are no support groups available in a person's area, the NHF can help interested persons start one.

National Institute of Neurological Disorders and
    Stroke (NINDS)
31 Center Drive MSC 2540
Building 31, Room 8A-06
Bethesda, MD 20892-2540
(800) 352-9424
Web site: http://www.ninds.nih.gov
e-mail: nindswebadmin@nih.gov
An agency of the United States federal government, this organization is the leading supporter of bio-medical research on the brain and nervous system.

In Canada

Migraine Association of Canada
365 Bloor Street, Suite 1912
Toronto, ON M4W 3L4
(416) 920-4916
(800) 663-3557
Web site: http://www.migraine.ca/index.htm
The Migraine Association publishes a quarterly newsletter, *Headlines,* and offers telephone counseling, referrals, and information on self-help groups. It aims to increase public awareness of migraine, sponsors Migraine Awareness Month every November, and encourages research for a cure for migraines.

Web Sites

Migraine Resource Center
http://www.migrainehelp.com
This site is sponsored by GlaxoWellcome, a pharmaceutical company. It provides information on migraine triggers as well as treatments and other information.

Ronda's Migraine Page
http://www.migrainepage.com
Maintained by Ronda Solberg, a migraine sufferer, this site offers tips and advice, links to other sources of help, and information from others with migraines.

For Further Reading

Albright, Peter, M.D. *The Complete Book of Complementary Therapies: The Best Known Alternative Therapies to Relieve Everyday Ailments.* Allentown, PA: People's Medical Society, 1997.

Cady, Roger, M.D., and Kathleen Farmer. *Headache Free: A Personalized Program to Stop Migraine, Cluster, Sinus, Tension, Menstrual, and Rebound Headaches.* New York: Bantam Books, 1996.

Cassileth, Barrie R. *The Alternative Medicine Handbook: The Complete Reference Guide to Alternative and Complementary Therapies.* New York: W.W. Norton & Company, 1998.

Diamond, Seymour, M.D. *The Hormone Headache: New Ways to Prevent, Manage, and Treat Migraine and Other Headaches.* New York: Macmillan, 1995.

Elkind, Arthur, M.D. *Migraines: Everything You Need to Know About Their Cause and Cure.* New York: Avon Books, 1997.

Gottlieb, Bill (ed.). *New Choices in Natural Healing: Over 1,800 of the Best Self-Help Remedies from the World of Alternative Medicine.* Emmaus, PA: Rodale Press, 1997.

Rapoport, Alan, M.D., and Fred Sheftell, M.D. *Conquering Headache.* Hamilton, Canada: Empowering Press, 1998.

Robbins, Lawrence, M.D., and Susan S. Lang. *Headache Help: A Complete Guide to Understanding Headaches and the Medicines That Relieve Them.* New York: Houghton Mifflin Company, 1995.

Votava, Andrea. *Coping With Migraines and Other Headaches.* New York: Rosen Publishing Group, 1997.

Index

A

alcohol, 26, 32
allergic reaction, 18
alternative treatments, 54–55
altitude headaches, 26
aneurysm, 25
angiography, 34
aura, 12, 17

B

basilar artery migraine, 14
biofeedback, 44–45
blood pressure, 26, 49
brain tumor, 19, 23–24, 54
breathing, conscious, 43–44

C

chronic tension headaches, 23
cluster headaches, 17

D

depression, 12, 28, 30–31
diagnostic tools, 33–34
diary, headache, 36–37
dizziness, 10, 14, 17

E

electroencephalogram (EEG), 34
episodic tension headaches, 22–23
exertional headaches, 25–26

G

genetics, 16, 17

I

imagery/visualization, 42–43
International Headache Society, 12

M

medications, 48–49, 50–52
meningitis, 24–25
migraines
    causes of, 17–18
    myths about, 18–19
    types of, 14–17
migraine equivalent, 10
MRI and MRA, 34

N

National Headache Foundation, 54
natural remedies, 47, 53
nausea, 7, 10, 51
neurologist, 30–31

P

prevention, 38–49
prodrome, 11

Q

questions, asked by doctors,
    12–14

S

sensitivity to lights and noise, 8, 22
serotonin, 18
severe head injury, 25
sinus, 18
specialists, 30–31
stress, avoiding, 41–42
subdural bleeding, 25
substances, 26
support groups, 54

T

t'ai chi chuan, 46, 47
tension headaches, 20–23
thunderclap headache, 25
treatment, 50–55
triggers, 10, 21, 32, 38–41

V

vertigo, 10, 14
vision, problems with, 14, 16, 17
vomiting, 7, 10, 14, 51

About the Author

Barbara Moe has master's degrees in nursing and social work. She has written several other books for the Rosen Publishing Group, including *Coping with Chronic Illness, Coping with Eating Disorders, Coping with Tic Disorders and Tourette's Syndrome, Understanding the Causes of a Negative Body Image, Everything You Need to Know About PMS,* and *Everything You Need to Know About Sexual Abstinence.* Ms. Moe used to suffer from migraine headaches.

Photo Credits

Cover by Darren Turner; pp. 2, 7, 15, 22, 27, 29, 43, 45, 51 by Kristen Artz; p. 9 © Reuters/Mike Segar/Archive Photos; p. 47 © Dean Conger/CORBIS; p. 13 © The Everett Collection; p. 24 © T. Youssef/Custom Medical Stock Photo; p. 35 © Science Photo Library/Custom Medical.